MATHEMATICS IN THF WAI

DRUG CALCULATIONS

SUSAN PIRIE
PETER SULLIVAN

Stanley Thornes (Publishers) Ltd

First published in 1984 by:
Stanley Thornes (Publishers) Ltd
Old Station Drive
Leckhampton
CHELTENHAM GL53 0DN
England

British Library Cataloguing in Publication Data

Pirie, Susan
    Mathematics in the ward: drug dosage calculations.
    1. Pharmaceutical arithmetic   2. Drugs—Dosage
    3. Nursing
    I. Title   II. Sullivan, P.
    615'.4'01513   RS57

ISBN 0-85950-367-4

Typeset by Tech-Set, Gateshead, Tyne & Wear
in 10/12 Helvetica
Printed and bound in Great Britain by
Swindon Press Limited, Swindon

This book was produced as a result of a visit by Susan Pirie to Papua New Guinea, sponsored by the British Council and the University of Technology, Lae. It was, therefore, written primarily for Papua New Guinean nurses, but will undoubtedly be useful wherever nurses are struggling to calculate drug doses, particularly in tropical or sub-tropical climates.

A

INTRODUCTION

Giving drugs to patients is a part of the everyday life of a practising nurse, and you probably have little difficulty working out the required doses of the common drugs in use on your ward.

Problems could arise, however, if you moved to a ward dealing with specialised drugs such as those used in cancer therapy, or if a new doctor prescribed drugs in an unfamiliar way. An even greater danger lies with the familiar drugs, because the suppliers sometimes alter the strength of their medications. You must be aware of this and know how to calculate the new dosage.

FORTUNATELY calculating drug doses can be simple, as you will see.

EXAMPLES

Consider the following example:

A1   A doctor prescribes 600 mg of aspirin p.r.n. Aspirin is available as tablets, each containing 300 mg.

You need to work out how many tablets the patient needs.

He needs 2 tablets — **EASY!**

Now look at a less familiar example:

A2   The doctor prescribes 24 mg of Vallergan. Vallergan forte syrop is available as 30 mg per 5 ml.

You need to work out how many millilitres to give the patient.

1

Not at all easy!

BUT . . . when you have worked through this book, you will be able to do this calculation with confidence.

There is one simple rule which will enable you to calculate **ANY** dose of **ANY** drug, however unfamiliar.

To do any drug calculation you need to know three things:

1 What has the doctor prescribed? —— What do you **WANT?**

2 What dose is available? —— What do you **HAVE?**

3 How is the dose 'packaged'? —— What is the **AMOUNT?**

In Example **A1**

The doctor prescribed 600 mg aspirin —— You **WANT** 600 mg.

The available dose is 300 mg —— You **HAVE** 300 mg.

The 'package' is 1 tablet —— The **AMOUNT** is 1 tablet.

In Example **A2**

The doctor prescribed 24 mg Vallergan —— You **WANT** 24 mg.

The available dose is 30 mg —— You **HAVE** 30 mg.

The 'package' is 5 ml —— The **AMOUNT** is 5 ml.

Now look at the following case history:

Naomi Bage is a 4-year-old child who came into hospital very sick and severely undernourished. She weighed only 10 kg. The doctor wrote up the drug sheet as follows:

Folic Acid 5 mg oral daily							
Streptomycin 250 mg IM daily							
Isoniazid 200 mg oral daily							
Chloramphenicol 250 mg oral q.i.d.							
Quinine 120 mg IM b.d.							

The drug cupboard contained:

Add 1.5 ml
sterile water
to make 2 ml
solution.

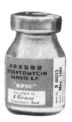

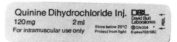

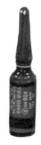

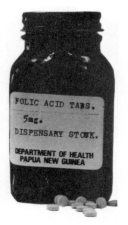

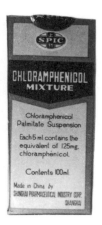

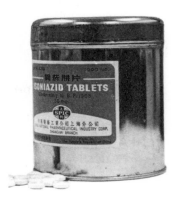

QUESTIONS

ANSWER THESE QUESTIONS BUT DO NOT CALCULATE THE DOSE YET

A3 Consider folic acid.

What has been prescribed?   What do you WANT?
What is available?   What do you HAVE?
How is the drug 'packaged'?   What is the AMOUNT?

CHECK YOUR ANSWERS

A4 Consider streptomycin.

What do you WANT? (Prescribed)
What do you HAVE? (Available)
What is the AMOUNT? ('Package')

A5 Consider isoniazid.

What do you WANT?
What do you HAVE?
What is the AMOUNT?

A6 Consider chloramphenicol.

What are the values for:
WANT?
HAVE?
AMOUNT?

A7 Consider quinine.

What are the values for:
WANT?
HAVE?
AMOUNT?

CHECK YOUR ANSWERS

Now consider the following prescriptions:

NAME: Kone Anis	NAME: Peter Kobu
10 mg folic acid I.M.	Ampicillin-500mg

NAME: Idan Mika	NAME: John Malu
125 mg Aminophylline I.V.	900 000 u Procaine Penicillin

The drug cupboard contained:

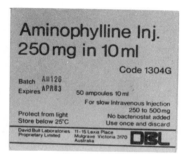

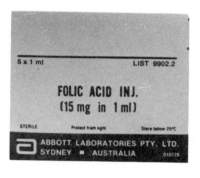

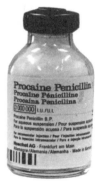

Add 10 ml
sterile water
to get 13 ml
solution.

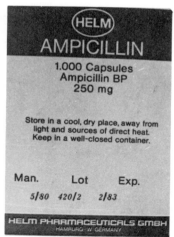

QUESTIONS

ANSWER THESE QUESTIONS BUT DO NOT CALCULATE THE DOSE YET

A8   Consider the prescription for Kone.

What do you WANT?
What do you HAVE?
What is the AMOUNT?

A9   Consider the prescription for Peter.

What do you WANT?
What do you HAVE?
What is the AMOUNT?

A10 Consider the prescription for Idan.

What do you WANT?
What do you HAVE?
What is the AMOUNT?

A11 Consider the prescription for John.

What do you WANT?
What do you HAVE?
What is the AMOUNT?

CHECK YOUR ANSWERS

B

THE RULE

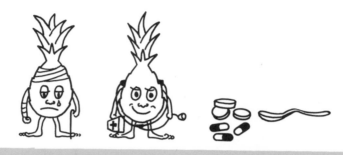

$$\text{DOSE} = \frac{\text{WANT}}{\text{HAVE}} \times \text{AMOUNT}$$

EXAMPLES

B1   Look at Example **A1** (page 2).

The doctor prescribed 600 mg of aspirin → **WANT** = 600 mg

The aspirin tablets contain 300 mg   → **HAVE** = 300 mg

The 'package' is 1 tablet   → **AMOUNT** = 1 tablet

The RULE gives:

$$\text{DOSE} = \frac{\text{WANT}}{\text{HAVE}} \times \text{AMOUNT}$$

$$= \frac{600 \text{ mg}}{300 \text{ mg}} \times 1 \text{ tablet}$$

$$= \underline{2 \text{ tablets}}$$

Is this the same answer as we had in Example **A1**?

B2 Now look back at Naomi Bage's drug sheet (page 3).

What dose of folic acid would you give her?

The RULE gives:

$$DOSE = \frac{WANT}{HAVE} \times AMOUNT$$

So $DOSE = \dfrac{5 \text{ mg}}{5 \text{ mg}} \times 1 \text{ tablet}$

$$= \underline{1 \text{ tablet}}$$

Do you agree?

QUESTIONS

B3 Look at Naomi's drug sheet again (page 3).

What dose of isoniazid would you give her?
Now calculate the dose using the RULE.
Do you get the same answer in both cases?

B4 Look at Naomi's sheet again.

What dose of quinine would you give her?
Do you get the same answer using the RULE?

C

CALCULATIONS

The exercises that you have just done were straightforward, but this type of calculation can be more complicated. This section gives you practice at the types of calculation that you may meet.

When you have numbers written this way: $\dfrac{120}{240}$ you need to be able to cancel in order to work out the answer. You may choose any number which divides exactly into the number on the bottom and the number on top.

EXAMPLE

C1
$$\frac{\overset{12}{\cancel{120}}}{\underset{24}{\cancel{240}}}$$
CANCEL BY 10

You can cancel again

$$\frac{\overset{6}{\cancel{\overset{12}{\cancel{120}}}}}{\underset{12}{\cancel{\underset{24}{\cancel{240}}}}}$$
CANCEL BY 2

and again

$$\frac{\overset{1}{\cancel{\overset{6}{\cancel{\overset{12}{\cancel{120}}}}}}}{\underset{2}{\cancel{\underset{12}{\cancel{\underset{24}{\cancel{240}}}}}}}$$
CANCEL BY 6   to get $\dfrac{1}{2} = \underline{0.5}$

QUESTIONS

Cancel the following:

C2 $\dfrac{250}{500}$ **C5** $\dfrac{225}{300}$

C3 $\dfrac{180}{90}$ **C6** $\dfrac{25}{125}$

C4 $\dfrac{60}{15}$ **C7** $\dfrac{144}{36}$

If you have 3 numbers written like this: $\dfrac{55}{330} \times 3$ you should first

rewrite it as: $\dfrac{55}{330} \times \dfrac{3}{1}$.

You may then cancel the numbers on the bottom with EITHER of the numbers on the top.

EXAMPLE

C8 $\dfrac{55}{330} \times 3 = \dfrac{55}{\cancel{330}} \times \dfrac{\cancel{3}^{1}}{1}$ CANCEL BY 3

$$\underset{110}{}$$

cancel again

$$\dfrac{\overset{5}{\cancel{55}}}{\underset{\underset{10}{\cancel{110}}}{\cancel{330}}} \times \dfrac{\overset{1}{\cancel{3}}}{1}$$ CANCEL BY 11

and again

$$\dfrac{\overset{1}{\cancel{\overset{5}{\cancel{55}}}}}{\underset{\underset{\underset{2}{\cancel{10}}}{\cancel{110}}}{\cancel{330}}} \times \dfrac{\overset{1}{\cancel{3}}}{1}$$ CANCEL BY 5   to get

$$\dfrac{1}{2} \times \dfrac{1}{1} = \dfrac{1}{2} = \underline{0.5}$$

QUESTIONS

Calculate the following:

C9 $\dfrac{150}{125} \times 5$

C12 $\dfrac{250}{75} \times 6$

C10 $\dfrac{500}{2000} \times 8$

C13 $\dfrac{500}{250} \times 3$

C11 $\dfrac{24}{30} \times 5$

C14 $\dfrac{75}{100} \times 2$

Most of the calculations a nurse does, involve cancelling by 10, 5 or 2.

You can cancel by 10 if a top AND a bottom number end in 0.

You can cancel by 5 if a top AND a bottom number end in 0 or 5.

You can cancel by 2 if a top AND a bottom number are even, that means they end in 2, 4, 6, 8 or 0.

You may not always be able to cancel all the numbers and you will have to finish with a division sum.

EXAMPLE

C15 $\dfrac{350}{400} \times 10 = \dfrac{\overset{35}{\cancel{350}}}{\underset{\underset{4}{\cancel{40}}}{\cancel{400}}} \times \dfrac{\overset{1}{\cancel{10}}}{1} = \dfrac{35}{4} = \underline{8.75}$

$$
\begin{array}{r}
8.75 \\
4\overline{)35.00} \\
\underline{32} \\
30 \\
\underline{28} \\
20 \\
\underline{20}
\end{array}
$$

11

QUESTIONS

Calculate the following:

C16 $\dfrac{120}{150} \times 3$ **C17** $\dfrac{35}{50} \times 5$ **C18** $\dfrac{90}{120} \times 5$

Sometimes the division does not give an exact answer, and you need to stop dividing somewhere. You cannot measure more accurately than 1 decimal place, so stop dividing when you have 2 decimal places in the answer and 'round off'.

ROUND OFF means:

If the number in the 2nd decimal place is 0, 1, 2, 3, 4 then ignore it.

If the number in the 2nd decimal place is 5, 6, 7, 8, 9 then add 1 to the number in the 1st decimal place.

For example

$\left.\begin{array}{l} 8.70 \\ 8.71 \\ 8.72 \\ 8.73 \\ 8.74 \end{array}\right\}$ round off to 8.7 $\left.\begin{array}{l} 8.75 \\ 8.76 \\ 8.77 \\ 8.78 \\ 8.79 \end{array}\right\}$ round off to 8.8

EXAMPLE

C19 $\dfrac{350}{600} \times 10 = \dfrac{\overset{35}{\cancel{350}}}{\underset{6}{\cancel{600}}} \times \dfrac{\overset{1}{\cancel{10}}}{1} = \dfrac{35}{6}$

$= \underline{5.8}$

$$\begin{array}{r} 5.83 \\ 6\overline{)35.00} \\ \underline{30} \\ 50 \\ \underline{48} \\ 20 \\ \underline{18} \\ \end{array}$$

STOP

round off to 5.8

12

QUESTIONS

Calculate the following:

C20 $\dfrac{140}{150} \times 5$ **C21** $\dfrac{50}{80} \times 2$ **C22** $\dfrac{500}{300} \times 5$

You can cancel even when the TOP number is a decimal, but you must be careful not to lose the decimal point.

EXAMPLES

C23 $\dfrac{12.5}{15} \times 3 = \dfrac{12.5}{\underset{5}{\cancel{15}}} \times \dfrac{\overset{1}{\cancel{3}}}{1}$ CANCEL BY 3

$= \dfrac{\overset{2.5}{\cancel{12.5}}}{\underset{\underset{1}{\cancel{5}}}{\cancel{15}}} \times \dfrac{\overset{1}{\cancel{3}}}{1}$ CANCEL BY 5   to get

$$\dfrac{2.5}{1} \times \dfrac{1}{1} = \underline{2.5}$$

C24 $\dfrac{2.5}{75} \times 2 = \dfrac{\overset{0.5}{\cancel{2.5}}}{\underset{15}{\cancel{75}}} \times \dfrac{2}{1}$ CANCEL BY 5

and again by 5

$\dfrac{\overset{\overset{0.1}{\cancel{0.5}}}{\cancel{2.5}}}{\underset{\underset{3}{\cancel{15}}}{\cancel{75}}} \times \dfrac{2}{1} = \dfrac{0.1}{3} \times \dfrac{2}{1} = \dfrac{0.2}{3}$

$= \underline{0.1}$

$$\begin{array}{r} 0.06 \\ 3\overline{)0.20} \\ \underline{18} \\ \text{STOP} \end{array}$$

Round off to 0.1

13

QUESTIONS

Calculate the following:

C25 $\dfrac{62.5}{250} \times 10$

C26 $\dfrac{12.5}{50} \times 7$

C27 $\dfrac{0.5}{50} \times 10$

D

USING THE RULE

EXAMPLES

D1   Mary Tau has been admitted recently to the Labour Ward, and is experiencing severe pains in the first stage of labour.

The doctor orders an injection of pethidine 75 mg IM.

Pethidine 75 mg IM				

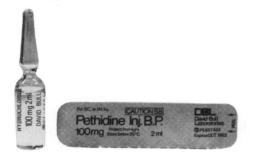

Pethidine is supplied in ampoules containing 100 mg in 2 ml of solution.

To calculate how much pethidine to draw up, we use the RULE:

$$DOSE = \frac{WANT}{HAVE} \times AMOUNT$$

Ask yourself these questions:

1   What do we WANT? ....   75 mg

2   What do we HAVE? ....   100 mg

3   What is the AMOUNT? ....   2 ml

So $\quad \text{DOSE} = \dfrac{75 \text{ mg}}{100 \text{ mg}} \times 2 \text{ ml}$ 1st CHECK: cancel the units

$$\text{DOSE} = \dfrac{75 \ \cancel{\text{mg}}}{100 \ \cancel{\text{mg}}} \times 2 \text{ ml}$$

This check ensures that you do not confuse the "HAVE" and the "AMOUNT". Notice also that the unit left, ml, is the unit of the answer.

Then we continue:

$$\text{DOSE} = \dfrac{75}{100} \times 2 \text{ ml}$$

$$= \dfrac{150}{100} \text{ ml}$$

$$= 1.5 \text{ ml}$$

2nd CHECK: compare the prescription with the ampoule. Since 75 mg is less than 100 mg, the answer must be less than 2 ml

D2 When a patient with malaria is not responding to chloroquine treatment, it may mean that it is the particular strain of malaria parasites which are resistant to chloroquine.

For one such case, the doctor ordered 350 mg of quinine to be given, deep in the buttock.

Quinine is available in an ampoule which contains 600 mg in 10 ml of solution.

You must calculate how much solution must be drawn up for this injection.

> CAUTION S4
>
> Supply of this preparation except on prescription is illegal
> KEEP OUT OF REACH OF CHILDREN
> 50 Ampoules each 10 ml
> **QUININE DIHYDROCHLORIDE 600 mg**
> FOR INTRAMUSCULAR INJECTIONS ONLY
> Each 10 ml ampoule contains
> 600 mg Quinine Dihydrochloride
> WARNING: Protect from light and store in a cool place
> Date of Manufacture: 12-80
> Batch No. 011145
> Expiry: 3 years
> **Drug Houses of Australia (Asia) Pte Ltd**
> Singapore

We use the RULE:

$$DOSE = \frac{WANT}{HAVE} \times AMOUNT$$

1   What do you WANT? .... 350 mg

2   What do you HAVE?........................ 600 mg

3   What is the AMOUNT? .... 10 mg

So   DOSE $= \dfrac{350 \text{ mg}}{600 \text{ mg}} \times 10$ ml

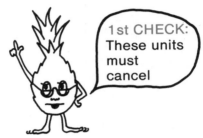

1st CHECK: These units must cancel

$$= \frac{\overset{35}{\cancel{350}}}{\underset{\underset{6}{\cancel{60}}}{\cancel{600}}} \times \overset{1}{\cancel{10}} \text{ ml}$$

$= \underline{5.8 \text{ ml}}$ 2nd CHECK: 350 mg is less than than 600 mg so dose must be less than 10 ml

QUESTIONS

D3   The doctor orders 150 mg 'O' chloramphenicol suspension for a patient with typhoid.

Chloramphenicol is labelled 125 mg in 5 ml.

Copy and complete the following:

1   WANT   =

2   HAVE   =

3   AMOUNT =

4   $DOSE = \dfrac{WANT}{HAVE} \times AMOUNT =$

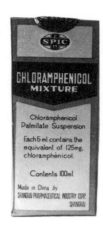

D4   A patient is admitted to hospital with pneumonia. The doctor prescribes 500 mg of tetracycline to be given. Tetracycline is available as shown. Explain how you will make up the correct dose.

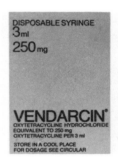

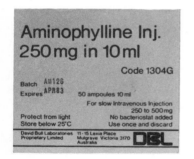

D5   A young girl, Betty, is diagnosed as having asthma. She is prescribed 62.5 mg of aminophylline IVI. It is available as shown.

What dose is required?

D6   Chloral hydrate is a sedative which induces a natural sleep quickly. 5 ml of solution contains 150 mg chloral hydrate. If the doctor orders 500 mg to be given, what is the necessary dose?

D7   You can now calculate the answer to Example **A2** (page 1). Try it.

E

FURTHER CALCULATIONS

EXAMPLES

E1   When you multiply by 10, the decimal point moves 1 place to the right:

$$2.5 \times 10 = 2\underset{\text{1 move}}{{}_{\circ}5} = 25$$

E2   When you multiply by 100, the decimal point moves 2 places to the right:

$$7.35 \times 100 = 7\underset{\text{2 moves}}{{}_{\circ}3\ 5} = 735$$

E3   When you multiply by 1000, the decimal point moves 3 places to the right:

$$0.625 \times 1000 = 0\underset{\text{3 moves}}{{}_{\circ}6\ 2\ 5} = 625$$

E4   If there are not enough numbers when you move the decimal point, you will have to write an extra 0.

$$8.22 \times 1000 = 8\underset{\substack{\text{3 moves need} \\ \text{an extra 0}}}{{}_{\circ}2\ 2\ 0} = 8220$$

QUESTIONS

Calculate the following:

E5 2.25×100 E8 0.025×10

E6 0.6×10 E9 1.2×1000

E7 3.8×100 E10 0.25×1000

19

Occasionally when you use the RULE:

$$DOSE = \frac{WANT}{HAVE} \times AMOUNT$$

you get something like: $\quad DOSE = \frac{6.6}{1.2} \times 2$

You MUST NOT cancel while there is a decimal on the bottom.

First you must MULTIPLY both the TOP and BOTTOM by 10, or 100, or 1000, to get a whole number on the bottom.

EXAMPLES

E11 $\quad \frac{6.6}{1.2} \times 2 = \frac{6.6 \times 10}{1.2 \times 10} \times \frac{2}{1} = \frac{6\,6.}{1\,2.} \times \frac{2}{1} = \frac{66}{12} \times \frac{2}{1}$

Now you may cancel

$$\frac{\overset{11}{\cancel{66}}}{\underset{6}{\cancel{12}}} \times \frac{\overset{1}{\cancel{2}}}{1} = \underline{11}$$

E12 $\quad \frac{0.5}{0.25} \times 1 = \frac{0.5 \times 100}{0.25 \times 100} \times 1 = \frac{0\,5\,0.}{0\,2\,5.} \times 1 = \frac{50}{25}$

Now you may cancel

$$\frac{\overset{2}{\cancel{50}}}{\underset{1}{\cancel{25}}} \times 1 = \underline{2}$$

QUESTIONS

Calculate the following:

E13 $\quad \frac{0.2}{1.2} \times 3$ **E15** $\quad \frac{1.4}{3.5} \times 2$ **E17** $\quad \frac{0.25}{0.5} \times 2$

E14 $\quad \frac{0.45}{0.6} \times 1$ **E16** $\quad \frac{1}{0.25} \times 5$ **E18** $\quad \frac{0.001}{0.05} \times 5$

F

WHEN THE UNITS ARE NOT THE SAME

You have seen in Section D that one of the very important CHECKS is to ensure the units cancel to leave only the units of the AMOUNT.

Consider the following example:

EXAMPLE

F1   Andrew Tabo is an 18-month-old child weighing only 7 kg. The doctor has diagnosed tuberculosis and written up his prescription as:

250 mg Streptomycin daily I.M.			
150 mg Isoniazid daily oral			

In the drug cupboard you have

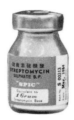

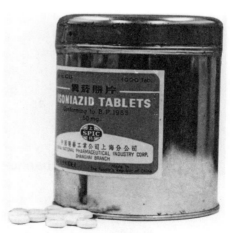

You calculate the isoniazid dose as follows:

WANT $= 150$ mg

HAVE $= 50$ mg

AMOUNT $= 1$ tablet

DOSE $= \dfrac{\text{WANT}}{\text{HAVE}} \times \text{AMOUNT}$

$ = \dfrac{150 \,\text{mg}}{50 \,\text{mg}} \times 1 \text{ tablet}$ 1st CHECK: cancel the units

$ = \underline{3 \text{ tablets}}$ 2nd CHECK: 150 mg is more than 50 mg so you need more than 1 tablet

EASY!

To calculate the streptomycin dose you must first add 1.5 ml sterile water to the vial. You then have 1 g in 2 ml. A table of dilutions is given on page 33.

DOSE $= \dfrac{\text{WANT}}{\text{HAVE}} \times \text{AMOUNT}$

WANT $= 250$ mg

HAVE $= 1$ g

AMOUNT $= 2$ ml

If you write $\dfrac{\text{WANT}}{\text{HAVE}}$ as $\dfrac{250 \text{ mg}}{1 \text{ g}}$ you cannot cancel the units.

So you must first change the 'HAVE' units to match the 'WANT' units.

1 g $= 1000$ mg

So HAVE $= 1000$ mg

22

then $\text{DOSE} = \dfrac{250\ \cancel{\text{mg}}}{1000\ \cancel{\text{mg}}} \times 2\ \text{ml}$ 1st CHECK: Cancel the units

$$= \frac{500}{1000}$$

$$= \underline{0.5\ \text{ml}}$$

2nd CHECK: 250 mg is much less than 1 g (1000 mg) so the answer should be much less than 2 ml

QUESTION

F2   A doctor diagnoses meningitis as the reason for Sara Mero's fever and headaches. He orders 750 mg chloramphenicol IM q.i.d.

Before calculating the drug dosage you need to add 4 ml sterile water to the vial to obtain 1 g chloramphenicol in 5 ml.

What do you WANT?

What do you HAVE?

What is the AMOUNT?

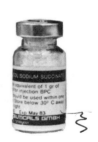

Use the RULE to calculate Sara's dose.

THINK ABOUT THE UNITS

DIGOXIN is a drug used in the treatment of heart conditions. It is dispensed as 500 μg in 2 ml.

'μg' stands for microgram. There are 1000 micrograms in 1 milligram (mg).

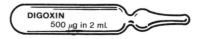

EXAMPLES

F3 A patient is prescribed 0.5 mg of digoxin IM. You need to calculate the dose to be given.

WANT   = 0.5 mg

HAVE   = 500 μg

AMOUNT = 2 ml

WANT and HAVE are not in the same units. Change WANT to micrograms.

0.5 mg   = 0.5 × 1000 μg

　　　　 = 500 μg

DOSE $= \dfrac{\text{WANT}}{\text{HAVE}} \times \text{AMOUNT}$

　　　　 $= \dfrac{500 \ \mu g}{500 \ \mu g} \times 2 \ ml$ 1st CHECK: cancel the units

　　　　 $= \underline{2 \ ml}$

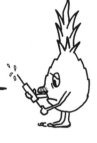

2nd CHECK: the dose prescribed equals the quantity of digoxin in the ampoule, so the whole ampoule should be given

When WANT and HAVE are not in the same units, it does not really matter which one you choose to change.

Look at Example **F3** again:

This time change HAVE to milligrams

500 μg = 500 ÷ 1000 mg = 0.5 mg

24

so   DOSE $= \dfrac{0.5 \text{ mg}}{0.5 \text{ mg}} \times 2 \text{ ml}$ 1st CHECK: cancel the units

You MUST NOT cancel when there is a decimal on the bottom.

First you must MULTIPLY both the TOP and BOTTOM by 10

$$\frac{0.5}{0.5} \times 2 \text{ ml} = \frac{0.5 \times 10}{0.5 \times 10} \times \frac{2}{1} \text{ ml}$$

$$= \frac{\overset{1}{\cancel{5}}}{\underset{1}{\cancel{5}}} \times \frac{2}{1} \text{ ml} \qquad \text{CANCEL BY 5}$$

$$= \underline{2 \text{ ml}}$$

The AMOUNT is exactly the same, whichever way you change the units.

Now look back at the streptomycin dose in Example **F1**:

WANT $= 250$ mg
HAVE $=$ 1 g
AMOUNT $=$ 2 ml

This time change WANT to grams

250 mg $= 250 \div 1000 \text{ g} = 0.25 \text{ g}$

DOSE $= \dfrac{0.25 \text{ g}}{1 \text{ g}} \times 2 \text{ ml}$ 1st CHECK: cancel the units

$= \underline{0.5 \text{ ml}}$

This is the same as the AMOUNT calculated on page 23.

It does NOT MATTER which units you change to, but you will always make the arithmetic easier if you change to the units which leave you with no decimals to work with.

PENICILLIN is dispensed in units (u).

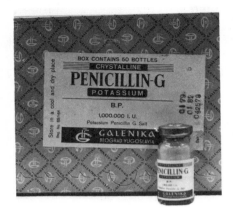

The doctor may write 1 000 000 u as 1 million u

> or 1×10^6 units

> or 1 Mega unit (Mu)
> (Mega simply means million)

10^6 means $10 \times 10 \times 10 \times 10 \times 10 \times 10 = 1\ 000\ 000$

1×10^6 means $1 \times 10 \times 10 \times 10 \times 10 \times 10 \times 10 = 1\ 000\ 000$

3×10^6 means $3 \times 10 \times 10 \times 10 \times 10 \times 10 \times 10 = 3\ 000\ 000$

1.25 Mega units means $1.25 \times 1\ 000\ 000$ units $= 1\overparen{2\ 5\ 0\ 0\ 0\ 0}$.
units

$= 1\ 250\ 000$
units

F4 Mary Gawi has severe septicaemia and is prescribed 2 Mega units of Crystapen. You must first add 2 ml sterile water to the vial to get 1 000 000 u in 2 ml.

WANT $= 2$ Mega units (Mu)

HAVE $= 1\ 000\ 000$ units (u)

AMOUNT $= 2$ ml

WANT and HAVE do not have the same units. Change WANT to units.

$$2\ Mu = 2 \times 1\ 000\ 000\ u = 2\ 000\ 000\ u$$

$$\text{DOSE} = \frac{\text{WANT}}{\text{HAVE}} \times \text{AMOUNT}$$

$$= \frac{2\,000\,000\,u}{1\,000\,000\,u} \times 2 \text{ ml}$$ 1st CHECK: cancel the units

$$= 2 \times 2 \text{ ml}$$ 2nd CHECK: 2 000 000 is
more than 1 000 000 so the
dose will be more than 2 ml

$$= \underline{4 \text{ ml}}$$

QUESTIONS

F5 A patient is prescribed 0.25 mg digoxin. Digoxin is available in an ampoule with 500 μg in 2 ml. What dose would you give?

F6 Procaine-amide injection, for a patient suffering from hypertension, comes in a vial containing 1 g in 10 ml. If the prescription says, "500 mg very slow IV". What dose would you give?

F7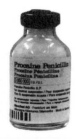

900 000 units of procaine penicillin IMI daily for 5 days is written up for Noka to treat her pneumonia.

What dose would you give her?

(Add 10 ml sterile water to give 13 ml solution.)

F8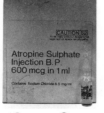

Gutuma, a 7-year-old child weighing 22 kg, is going for surgery. The doctor has prescribed 0.45 mg atropine sulphate as a premedication.

What dose would you give her?

F9

"1500 mg of potassium chloride to be added to each litre of 4% dextrose in $\frac{1}{5}$ normal saline" is written up for Ranu who has diarrhoea.

What dose would you give her?

G

DOSE PER KILOGRAM

Some drugs are prescribed according to body weight. This means that you must first calculate "what you WANT", depending on the patient's weight.

EXAMPLE

G1   A patient, Mana, is admitted to hospital with suspected malaria. A blood slide test is positive, but he is vomiting and is dehydrated. His weight is 46 kg.

The doctor orders chloroquine injection, IM at a rate of 4 mg per kg of body weight.

The injection is supplied as 80 mg in 2 ml.

FIRST calculate what you WANT.

Since Mana weighs 46 kg and the doctor orders 4 mg for each kilogram, we must multiply 46 by 4 to get WANT.

So WANT = 46 × 4

> You must multiply the dose per kg by the patient's weight to find the value of WANT

= 184 mg

Then continue as before:

HAVE   = 80 mg

AMOUNT = 2 ml

28

So $\text{DOSE} = \dfrac{\text{WANT}}{\text{HAVE}} \times \text{AMOUNT}$

$\dfrac{184 \text{ mg}}{80 \text{ mg}} \times 2 \text{ ml}$ 1st CHECK: cancel the units

$= \dfrac{368}{80}$

$= \underline{4.6 \text{ ml}}$ 2nd CHECK: 184 mg is more than 80 mg so you need more than 2 ml

QUESTIONS

G2 A doctor prescribes 4 mg/kg chloroquine injection for a patient who weighs 35 kg. Chloroquine injection is available as 80 mg in 2 ml. How much solution must be drawn up for the injection?

G3 Diphenhydramine elixir is an antihistamine for children, suitable for treating certain allergies. It is available as 10 mg in every 5 ml. A doctor orders 1 mg/kg for a child who weighs 12.5 kg. What is the required dose?

G4 Promethazine is a strong sedative and is available as 25 mg in 1 ml injection. If the doctor prescribes 0.5 mg/kg IM, what will be the dose for a child who weighs 20 kg?

G5 Diazepam injection (Valium) is available as 10 mg in 2 ml of solution. The dose for children is 0.5 mg/kg of body weight. How much should be drawn up for a patient who weighs 17 kg?

H

INSULIN

INSULIN is a drug given to patients suffering from diabetes. Insulin is not as yet very frequently used in Papua New Guinea. The dose of insulin prescribed varies widely from patient to patient, and for this reason several strengths of insulin are available.

BUT . . . all insulin calculations can be done using the RULE.

Insulin is manufactured in the following strengths:

40 units/ml (u/ml)

80 units/ml

20 units/ml

100 units/ml

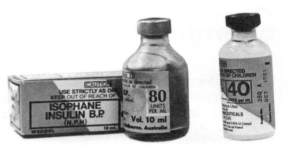

At present 40 units/ml and 80 units/ml are the most commonly available strengths.

EXAMPLES

H1   Vano Tago has been prescribed a daily dose of 50 units of insulin. If only insulin strength 40 u/ml is available then:

WANT   = 50 u

HAVE   = 40 u

AMOUNT = 1 ml

So $DOSE = \dfrac{WANT}{HAVE} \times AMOUNT = \dfrac{50\ u}{40\ u} \times 1$ ml

1st CHECK: cancel the units

$= \underline{1.25\text{ ml of }40\text{ strength}}$

2nd CHECK: 50 units is more than 40 units so the dose will be more than 1 ml.

H2 If only insulin strength 80 u/ml is available, then what dose would you give Vano?

WANT $= 50$ u

HAVE $= 80$ u

AMOUNT $= 1$ ml

So $DOSE = \dfrac{WANT}{HAVE} \times AMOUNT$

$= \dfrac{50\ u}{80\ u} \times 1$ ml   1st CHECK: cancel the units

$= \underline{0.625\text{ ml of }80\text{ strength}}$ 2nd CHECK: units is less than 80 units so less than 1 ml is needed

Look at the two answers:

1.25 ml of 40 strength (40 u/ml)

0.625 ml of 80 strength (80 u/ml)

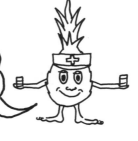

COMPARISON CHECK: 40 strength is weaker than 80 strength, so Vano needs more of the weak insulin

QUESTIONS

H3 Suppose only insulin strength 20 u/ml is available for Vano.

What do you WANT?
What do you HAVE?
What is the AMOUNT?
Use the RULE to calculate Vano's dose of 20 strength insulin.
Compare your answer with the doses given in Examples **H1** and **H2**.

H4 Calculate the dose of insulin strength 100 u/ml needed by Vano.
Compare your answer with one of the other insulin doses for Vano.

H5 Ela Tano is a diabetic who needs 20 units of insulin daily. Calculate her dose of 40 strength (40 u/ml) insulin.

H6 Calculate Ela's insulin dose if only 80 strength is available. Compare your answers to **H5** and **H6** with the doses given in Examples **H1** and **H2**.

DILUTIONS

Several times in this book drugs have been mentioned which need diluting before you can calculate the dose to give. Below is a list of drugs in common use. Space has been left for you to add any new drugs you wish to refer to:

TABLE OF DILUTIONS

Ampicillin 100 mg 200 mg 250 mg 500 mg	Add ½ ml 1 ml 1 ml 2 ml	To get 100 mg in ½ ml 200 mg in 1 ml 250 mg in 1 ml 500 mg in 2 ml
Chloramphenicol 1 g	Add 4 ml	To get 1 g in 5 ml
Penicillin, benzyl 1 Mu (Crystapen)	Add 2 ml	To get 1 000 000 u in 2 ml
Penicillin, procaine 3 Mu	Add 10 ml	To get 3 000 000 u in 13 ml
Streptomycin 1 g 5 g for neonates 1 g	Add 1.5 ml 7 ml 4.5 ml	To get 1 g in 2 ml 5 g in 10 ml 1 g in 5 ml
BCG vaccine 1 mg	Add 2 ml	To get 1 mg in 2 ml

On the previous page is a table of dilutions. The questions below will give you some practice in using the table. It would be a good idea to keep a copy of this table on the ward so that when you need to make a dilution you can check how much sterile water you need to add and what the AMOUNT will be.

EXAMPLE

I1   What must you add to chloramphenicol 1 g?   4 ml

What do you get? .... 1 g in 5 ml

What is the AMOUNT? .... 5 ml

QUESTIONS

I2   What must you add to ampicillin 250 mg?

What do you get?

What is the AMOUNT?

I3   What do you add to streptomycin 1 g for neonates?

What do you get?

What is the AMOUNT?

ANSWERS

SECTION A

	WANT =		HAVE =		AMOUNT =	
A3	WANT =	5 mg	HAVE =	5 mg	AMOUNT =	1 tablet
A4	=	250 mg	=	1 g	=	2 ml
A5	=	200 mg	=	50 mg	=	1 tablet
A6	=	250 mg	=	125 mg	=	5 ml
A7	=	120 mg	=	120 mg	=	2 ml
A8	WANT =	10 mg	HAVE =	15 mg	AMOUNT =	1 ml
A9	=	500 mg	=	250 mg	=	1 capsule
A10	=	125 mg	=	250 mg	=	10 ml
A11	=	900 000 u	=	3 000 000 u	=	13 ml

SECTION B

B3	4 tablets
B4	2 ml

SECTION C

C2	$\frac{1}{2} = 0.5$		C20	4.7
C3	2		C21	1.3
C4	4		C22	8.3
C5	$\frac{3}{4} = 0.75$		C25	2.5
C6	$\frac{1}{5} = 0.2$		C26	1.8
C7	4		C27	0.1
C9	6			
C10	2			
C11	4			
C12	20			
C13	6			
C14	1.5 or 1½			
C16	2.4			
C17	3.5			
C18	3.75 or 3.8			

SECTION D

D3	150 mg, 125 mg, 5 ml, 6 ml
D4	6 ml or 2 syringes
D5	2.5 ml
D6	16.7 ml
D7	4 ml

SECTION E

E5	225	**E13**	½ or 0.5
E6	6	**E14**	0.8
E7	380	**E15**	0.8
E8	0.25	**E16**	20
E9	1200	**E17**	1
E10	250	**E18**	0.1

SECTION F

F2   750 mg, 1 g = 1000 mg, 5 ml, 3.75 ml
F5   1 ml
F6   5 ml
F7   3.9 ml
F8   0.75 ml
F9   6 ml

SECTION G

G2   3.5 ml
G3   6.25 ml
G4   0.4 ml
G5   1.7 ml

SECTION H

H3   50 u, 20 u, 1 ml, 2.5 ml
H4   0.5 ml
H5   0.5 ml
H6   0.25 ml

SECTION I

I2   1 ml, 250 mg in 1 ml, 1 ml
I3   4.5 ml, 1 g in 5 ml, 5 ml

The correct calculation of drug doses is obviously critical in medical and nursing practice, and for special reasons is in certain circumstances a complex process.

Dr Pirie's little book was written primarily for use by nurses in Papua New Guinea, but will be particularly useful wherever nurses are struggling to calculate drug doses in tropical or sub-tropical climates.

Stanley Thornes

Old Station Drive
Leckhampton
CHELTENHAM
Glos. GL53 0DN

ISBN 0-85950-367-4

9 780859 503679